TOTAL
reflexology

TOTAL
reflexology

Everything you need to unlock the healing power of your body

Kevin and Barbara Kunz

BARNES & NOBLE

NEW YORK

Contents

Introduction

WELCOME TO TOTAL REFLEXOLOGY!

Your health in your hands—and in your feet! Hand and foot reflexology has provided positive steps toward better health for the millions of people around the world who use it daily. Reflexology techniques apply pressure to the feet and hands, nourishing the body with soothing signals. Whether you're using hands-on techniques or self-help tools such as the foot roller or reflex ball, the pressure you're creating will give you a feel-good feeling. And feeling good is something you can practice!

Triggering the positive impacts of reflexology is easily within reach. With creative and easy ways to interrupt stress, reflexology surrounds enthusiasts with opportunities to use its techniques throughout the day. By applying a systematic program of pressure techniques, you tap into pressure sensors in the hands and feet that act together with the entire body to enable us to move through the day. These same sensors contribute to the body's physical level of tension. Interrupt this tension enough and your body will revitalize itself. The successful reflexology experience allows you to take a break, resetting your body and providing a mini-vacation for your feet and hands.

Reflexology also provides the ability to target specific concerns, such as health problems or injuries. By tapping into the reflex areas on your hands and feet, you can become empowered to take charge of your body and the way you feel. The more you do, the bigger effect you'll have on your body.

Our client Jane, for example, had chronic asthma that caused her to wake up in the middle of the night unable to breathe, and she had become desensitized to most medications. We applied reflexology to Jane's hands and feet, focusing on the Lung reflex area, and gave her self-help tools she could use herself at home. Soon Jane could sleep through the night. Best of all, she was now in control of her own health, and could even use reflexology as a preventive measure against health problems for her two teenaged daughters. Jane's family's sense of well-being and quality of life was enhanced by low-cost, easy-to-use reflexology techniques.

You too can find health in your hands and in your feet . . . starting now!

REFLEXOLOGY HISTORY

Use of reflexology, often handed down from generation to generation, has grown into a tradition in countries around the world. Many of today's reflexology techniques and theories stem from time-honored traditions dating back to the dawn of time. While it may seem natural to rub a tired hand or stubbed toe, evidence points to reflexology work as a therapy utilized by ancient physicians. Egyptian pictographs dating from 2350 B.C.E. carved into stone at the Tomb of the Physician at Saqqara depict scenes representing a form of reflexology. In the Medical Teachers Temple at Nara, Japan, built in A.D. 790, bronze statues of seated Buddhas have special symbols cast into their hands and feet that are thought to reflect reflex areas. Chinese, Indian, and other ancient cultures show evidence of reflexology practices as well.

As it was handed down through the ages, reflexology use and techniques ebbed and flowed. Today's reflexology came about as physicians of the late 1800s were trying to explore how the nervous system worked by using needles, pressure, the application of heat or cold, vibrations, and other techniques. Their results came to be viewed as reflexes, which led to the development of stimulating reflex areas on the hands and feet to impact specific parts of the body. Reflexology was also gaining a foothold in Asia, where hands-on work, self-help tools, and cobblestone paths were all in common use by the late 1900s.

In ancient times, Octavian noted that Marc Anthony rubbed Cleopatra's feet at dinner parties. In the modern world, Princess Diana had foot reflexology three times a week. In 2004, her letters to her reflexologist sold at auction for £19,400 ($38,100).

In 1938, American physiotherapist Eunice Ingham was the first to fully develop and describe reflexology in a written work, *Stories the Feet Can Tell*, which outlined a system for applying pressure to the feet for expected health results. Many American and European hands-on reflexology systems resulted from Ingham's work, and more ideas have been incorporated into it over the years.

Today, people are drawn to reflexology use worldwide. Go shopping almost anywhere and you'll find pronged balls and sandals and electric hand and foot massagers. In Singapore, you can even see your own reflexologist at the reflexology kiosk at the mall. In Taiwan, tourists come from across Asia just for specific types of reflexology services that are offered by one of the region's many practitioners. China alone has more than five million reflexologists.

Parks in Asia are full of health-seekers walking on specially designed "reflexology paths," which simulate cobblestones and stimulate your feet when walked upon. So common are reflexology paths, hardly a condominium complex in Malaysia or Singapore is built without one. In Germany and Austria, reflexology paths are made with rocks, sticks, and mud. Cobblestone paths and portable cobblestone mats are becoming more and more popular in the United States, especially in the Northwest.

HOW REFLEXOLOGY WORKS

The pressure techniques of reflexology applied to the hands and feet trigger a relaxation response in the body. Triggering this relaxation response regularly throughout the day breaks up patterns of stress, and when these patterns are interrupted enough, the body is conditioned to function better. Like a successful exercise program, a successful reflexology style includes strategizing how often, how long, and how much technique is applied. As a user of reflexology, you will have to find the combination that works for you.

Reflexology's potential to relax the body and influence well-being is supported by scientific research. Some seventy controlled studies document positive results from reflexology work with disorders ranging from dysmenorrhea (discomfort during menstruation) to toothache. Positive effects have been experienced from all types of reflexology work, whether they're used on the hand or on the foot, done manually or with a tool, performed by another or practiced on yourself. Studies from around the world have shown proven results when using reflexology to improve digestion, help to regulate insulin in diabetics, help kidney function, lower blood pressure, lessen the pain and duration of childbirth, relieve the symptoms of chemotherapy, recover from surgery more quickly, and reduce spasms for multiple sclerosis patients. Reflexology has been shown to help ease depression and insomnia, and has even alleviated restlessness and wandering in Alzheimer's patients. Where you begin is up to you!

REFLEX AREAS

Reflex areas, shown on the charts, gloves, and socks in this kit, are targets for techniques. Getting to know the reflex areas will help you better obtain your health goals. Reflexology is the systematic, organized application of pressure techniques to the hands and feet, and the reflexology charts provide a map of where to apply these techniques to get results.

The reflexology socks and gloves will give you a good idea of where to find your reflex areas, but they should be used just as a guide. Use the laminated chart and your own experience to better pinpoint areas, some of which are minute.

The reflexology chart mirrors the body. The fingers and toes reflect the head and neck, while the heels correspond to the lower back. In between are the body's central organs and musculoskeletal structure. The left side of the body is mirrored on the left hand and foot, while the right side is reflected on the right hand and foot. As you go, pay attention to which parts of the hands and feet feel stressed, and see if this mirrors the corresponding parts of your body.

Look over the reflexology chart, sock, or glove. If the part of the body you'd like to affect is listed, this reflex area is your starting place for technique application. For more specific health concerns, see Chapter One: Reflex Areas. This chapter will give you specific techniques you can use to affect the relevant reflex areas on yourself or someone else. As you become more skillful at focusing the right technique on the right reflex area, you'll notice that it takes less time to be effective.

Bolster your efforts by also learning techniques for general relaxation. An overall sense of relaxation will advance your progress with a specific health concern. Overall sessions by someone else (which can be found in Chapter Four) provide even further relaxation. Consider trading sessions with a reflexology buddy or seeking professional services. Finally, supercharge your efforts by simply relaxing and enjoying the reflexology experience.

SETTING A GOAL

Just as a bite out of an apple is a step toward health, every application of reflexology's techniques takes a step as well. Focusing on a goal, however, will allow you to be better able to target your concern and get results.

Once you see results, you'll be motivated to do more reflexology. Success will breed success as you reach one health goal and move on to another.

Our asthmatic client Jane, for instance, had the goal of being free of the asthma attacks that would awake her during the night. After learning the simple self-help technique, Jane was able to control her attacks and breathe more easily within three minutes of applying it. Fortified by results, Jane increased her efforts by applying the technique throughout the day. Soon she had accomplished her goal.

As you choose a goal or goals, consider the following: Are you seeking to trigger an overall relaxation response, rejuvenate feet or hands, or focus on the health benefits of a reflex effect? If overall relaxation is your goal, you'll want to apply techniques to the whole foot or hand. If rejuvenating feet and hands is your goal, focus in on the areas that feel stressed. If you're seeking to impact a health concern, you'll want to target the relevant reflex areas. Once you've decided on a goal, decide to get yourself there!

For each technique in Chapters Two and Three, you'll find sidebars that give you specific instructions on how to use that technique to achieve your goals.

CHOOSING THE TECHNIQUES THAT ARE RIGHT FOR YOU

Set the stage for success by choosing the reflexology techniques that are right for you. The right technique matches you: the amount of effort you want to make, your available time, and your likes and dislikes. Self techniques, which include using the foot roller, reflex ball, and your own hands, can be found in Chapter Two. As you try out the techniques, keep the following in mind:

Experiment with combining different techniques and trying new tools to find the type of reflexology you like. Feel free to create a technique that works for you!

Do you like it? Follow your fancy: use a technique you like. A good indicator will be whether or not you are able to find the time and energy to do it. Choosing a technique that appeals to you will make you want to do it more often, allowing you to more easily work the technique into your routine and get results. Enjoying your reflexology work will also release the feel-good hormones that are beneficial to your body.

Does it match your energy level? Reflexology techniques should be relaxing, not taxing. In general, if you try a technique and it seems like a lot of work, it may not be the one for you. Pick a technique that matches your available effort. If you're tired after a long day, for example, you may want to choose a technique that requires less energy, such as one of the foot roller techniques.

Do you have the ability? Consider whether or not the chosen technique is within your level of ability. Some techniques require the foot to be placed in one's lap. Others call for some strength. If you're having trouble, go with your abilities to choose a technique that's right for you. Make sure to allow yourself time to learn new techniques. Reflexology use is both a physical activity and a life skill. It's worth the time investment to become proficient.

FINDING TIME

Just as with any exercise, you'll want to do reflexology enough to prompt a change. The more you apply reflexology techniques, the more you interrupt stress. The more you interrupt stress, the more you trigger the body's natural repair system. Frequency, duration, and intensity (how often, how long, and how much) are the keys to being successful in reflexology. Every time you apply pressure to your feet or your hands, you are creating positive change.

If finding time is a problem, try choosing a reflexology technique that you can do while doing something else, such as watching television, using the computer, commuting on mass transit, or traveling as a passenger in a car. Decide on possible opportunities in which you'd have time to use reflexology, and pick a technique that fits. For example, a foot roller technique is great for using under your desk at work.

Set up your reflexology possibilities in advance. Place your reflex ball or foot roller anywhere you may be with a few minutes of free time: at your easy chair, at your desk, in the glove compartment, or inside your handbag or briefcase. This worked well for our client Ed, who was plagued by pollens for years until he kept golf balls handy to use to affect his allergies.

Consider setting aside time to do reflexology every day. Ed, for example, used a reflex ball technique on his hands at each meal, three times a day. Get into the habit of integrating reflexology into your routine. Stack enough of these good habits together, and things will change for the better.

Using an electric tool such as a vibrating platform, a foot rolling machine, or a massaging wand can save you both time and effort. Results will be more generalized, but over time consistent use will lessen stress.

MAKING IT WORK

Getting results is all a matter of focused effort: your goal partnered with the right technique, the right reflex areas, and the right amount of time. Your reflexology success derives from a reflexology style that fits you. After you've determined what you want to accomplish, picked a technique, and found the opportunities to apply it, all you need to do is stick with it! More than anything else, regular technique application leads to successful use of reflexology.

In our more than twenty-five years of practice, we have noticed that it is those who do self-help or see their reflexologist regularly who see the biggest results. Being consistent with your reflexology program will not only help you maintain well-being, it will also help you when you need it most. Our thirteen-year-old niece was injured in a riding accident when her fingers were intertwined with the reins of a horse that took off running. Three fingers were in danger of paralysis, or even amputation. She credits the practice of daily self-help reflexology techniques throughout her convalescence with regaining the use of these fingers.

When reflexology becomes a part of your life, it's easy to recognize the possibilities of reflexology and remember to use it. Our client Jane, who had originally come to see us for asthma attacks, found herself in the emergency room with her daughter, who was experiencing extreme abdominal distress. For various medical reasons, no painkiller was administered during their five-hour wait for a diagnosis and operation, and Jane was able to draw on her reflexology experience to calculate where to press her daughter's hand to ease the pain.

APPROPRIATE USES OF REFLEXOLOGY

An important part of reflexology theory is deciding when to use reflexology and when not to use it. Never use reflexology techniques to work directly on a cut or bruise; any part of an injured hand, foot, wrist, or ankle; an ingrown nail; a rash; plantar warts or corns; split skin between toes or a cracked callus; athlete's foot; or any foot problem that requires the attention of a podiatrist.

Do not work on a reflex area that is overly sensitive, and make sure not to overwork a single part of the foot or hand. If a part of the foot or hand feels bruised or tender to the touch, it may be overworked. Let it rest for a few days. When you begin your work again, work lightly and for a shorter amount of time.

One can make an assessment of the stressed parts of the body using reflexology, but there is a difference between an assessment and a diagnosis. Never use reflexology to diagnose critical issues involving an individual's health. Reflexology provides input, but it should not constitute the basis for your actions. Follow standard first aid or a medically recommended response first.

Finally, self-help tools are just that: instruments used to work on oneself. Never use the foot roller, reflex ball, or another reflexology tool on someone else. There's no way to judge the impact of an instrument unless you yourself are receiving its impact.

AS YOU GO ALONG . . . USING REFLEXOLOGY

Both you and the recipient of your reflexology work will become adept at changing techniques to achieve the results you are seeking. As your work progresses, continually consider the effects it has. What exactly do you consider a benefit of your work? As one client commented, "I suddenly realized I could turn my head when driving to look at the traffic behind me." Effects can be subtle. Is the individual sleeping better? Do your shoes feel more comfortable? What other indicators of change can you see?

When applying techniques to yourself and others, use the socks and gloves to home in on reflex areas or to find out which parts of the body are stressed. For more sensitivity, remove the socks and gloves for an overall session.

You are seeking just the right ingredients to most effectively and efficiently get results. Which areas you are targeting, as well as how much pressure to apply, how long to apply pressure, and how frequently you are applying pressure, will vary from situation to situation. The right formula—how much pressure is used and how long to apply it—gets results. Here are some things to keep in mind as you go along:

Find the comfort zone. How much pressure you apply should always be within your comfort zone. Be aware of how the technique feels to you. You should be thinking, "That feels good." If there is a feeling of sensitivity, it should be a feeling of "it hurts good" rather than "it hurts bad." Discontinue work that "feels bad." If you're working on someone else, ask him or her "How does that feel?" as you go along and make sure you are working within his or her comfort level. If you aren't, ask, "Do you want me to go on?" When you proceed, make sure you proceed with respect for his or her comfort level.

If you are working on children, be aware that young children often do not have the words to express their reactions to your work or have the same response to pressure application that adults do. While an adult will respond with an expression of pain, a child will squirm as if to escape. (Some may leave at this point if you don't quickly soften your approach. Children are harsh critics.) When asked "Does that hurt?" they may say "No, it feels funny," or "No, it tickles."

Pick up the signals. It is a basic tenet of reflexology that pressing on the foot or hand will cause an effect throughout the body. It is also true, however, that in applying reflexology techniques to the foot or hand, you are applying pressure to a foot or hand! As you will probably notice, the person you are working on will react as you go through your reflexology session. In addition to asking your reflexology buddy how the technique feels, be aware of the nonverbal communication about your work. Keep an eye on the individual's face to gauge his or her reaction.

Get the "feel" of reflexology. As you work with the feet or the hands, consider what you're feeling under your working thumb or fingers. As you gain experience, you will also gain more and more of a sense of the "feel" for the surface of the hand or foot. The patterns of stress you feel will create target areas for technique application. You will notice the change in the way the surface feels as your work progresses or as stress factors enter you or the individual's life.

ACTIVATING THE REFLEXOLOGY LIFESTYLE

There are many uses for reflexology. For some, reflexology offers the opportunity to spend special time with a family member or friend. For others, reflexology provides potential help for a health concern or happier hands and feet. For still others, reflexology offers a full range of such uses as maintaining physical dexterity and walking abilities, overall relaxation, and preventing illness.

Whatever your plans for reflexology use, consider not only how to do reflexology but also how to make it a part of your lifestyle. Plan for success by exploring your options in regard to techniques, time, and available locations for practice. On the following pages, we will focus on popular and successful reflexology techniques and give you the tools to incorporate reflexology into your life. But the goal of this book is to help you find a reflexology style that works for you. Just as decorating a room allows for personal creativity and expression, your reflexology style is your own. Use this book to design your reflexology experience. Fun, easy ways to feel better with reflexology are at hand—and under foot!

Keep the laminated chart handy as you go through this book. It will show you the hand and foot charts that are a map to your body.

1

Reflex Areas

BECOMING EMPOWERED TO ACHIEVE YOUR HEALTH GOALS is one of the biggest benefits of reflexology. This section will not only give you a place to begin your reflexology work, it will better acquaint you with which parts of your feet and hands correspond to which parts of your body. After you find your health concern, use the diagrams at the top of that page along with the laminated chart and the socks and gloves to pinpoint which reflex area to home in on to achieve results. Areas on right side of your body will be reflected on the right foot and hand, and areas on the left side of your body will be reflected on the left foot and hand. Keep in mind, reflexology should never be used as a diagnostic tool. If a particular area feels stressed, it simply means that the corresponding part of the body may be in the need of relaxing, not that there is something wrong with it.

At the bottom of each page, you'll find techniques you can use to affect the desired reflex area. Techniques to use for yourself are shown in green, and techniques to use when giving someone else a reflexology session are shown in blue. After you find the technique that's right for you, apply it several times throughout the day to get results, and see your health improve.

ACNE

Acne, commonly known as pimples or zits, are lesions of the skin caused by clogged pores. Pores get clogged when too much oil is produced by the sebaceous (oil) glands, often caused by our hormones. Pimples are most typically found on the face, neck, back, chest, and shoulders. Although acne is usually not a serious health threat, it can be a source of significant emotional distress.

Reflex areas: Adrenal glands, Kidneys

FOOT TECHNIQUES

Foot roller on the middle
of your arch
(p. 107)

Thumb walk on the arch
(p. 146)

HAND TECHNIQUES

Reflex ball on heel of your
hand below the thumb
(p. 116)

Pinch technique on the
webbing between your
thumb and index finger
(p. 122)

Thumb walk on heel of the
hand below the thumb
(p. 154)

ALLERGIES

Allergies are an overreaction of the body's defense mechanisms. These defense mechanisms, which normally protect against infection, can be triggered by certain foods, clothing fibers, pollens, and other materials. Use these techniques to help combat the symptoms of allergies; with continued work, you may also become less allergy-prone. Note: for allergy symptoms, hand techniques tend to work better than foot techniques.

Reflex area: Adrenal glands

FOOT TECHNIQUES

Foot roller on the arch, angling your foot to the center, then to the outside (p. 106)

Thumb walk on the arch (p. 146)

HAND TECHNIQUES

Reflex ball on your
lower palm
(p. 116)

Single-finger grip on the
heel of your hand
below your thumb
(p. 121)

Single-finger grip on
the heel of the hand
below the thumb
(p. 132)

Thumb walk on the heel of
the hand below the thumb
(p. 153)

ANXIETY

At some time or another, we've all experienced anxiety—a feeling of apprehension, worry, uneasiness, or dread, oftentimes about a future event. Constant or unreasonable feelings of anxiety are considered anxiety disorders. Try using reflexology the next time you're feeling anxious.

Reflex area: Solar plexus

FOOT TECHNIQUES

Foot roller in between the
ball and arch of your foot
(p. 105)

Thumb walk between
the ball and arch
(p. 144)

HAND TECHNIQUES

Pinch technique below
your thumb and each
of your fingers
(p. 122)

Reflex ball at the base
of your thumb
(p. 115)

Thumb walk on
base of thumb
(p. 154)

Single-finger grip in the
webbing of the hand
(p. 131)

ARTHRITIS

Generally, arthritis is a painful inflammation of the joints. Depending on the type of arthritis, it can be a continuous ache or pain in certain areas when moving, and normally affects those over forty.

Reflex areas: Adrenal glands, Kidneys

FOOT TECHNIQUES

Foot roller on the middle
of your arch
(p. 107)

Thumb walk on the arch
(p. 146)

HAND TECHNIQUES

Reflex ball on heel of your
hand below the thumb
(p. 116)

Pinch technique on the
webbing between your
thumb and index finger
(p. 122)

Thumb walk on heel of the
hand below the thumb
(p. 154)

ASTHMA

Asthma is inflammation of the bronchial tubes that can make it hard to breathe. Associated with wheezing and coughing, asthma is often triggered by inhaling allergens such as pollen, mold spores, animal dander, or dust, and is the leading cause of chronic illness among children. Use reflexology to make asthma attacks less severe. Regular work in these areas can also help prevent severe bronchial tube inflammation (which leads to asthma attacks).

Reflex areas: Lungs, Adrenal glands

FOOT TECHNIQUES

Foot roller on the
ball of your foot
(p. 105)

Thumb walk on the
ball the foot
(p. 144)

Lung press dessert
(p. 164)

HAND TECHNIQUES

Reflex ball on the heel below your thumb (p. 116)

Single-finger grip technique on the heel below your thumb (p. 121)

Single-finger grip on the heel below the thumb (p. 132)

Thumb walk on the heel below the thumb (p. 153)

BACK PAIN

Most of us have suffered from back pain at some point or another. To use reflexology to help ease a sore back or combat postural fatigue, focus your reflexology work on the spine, the support structure for our bodies.

Reflex area: Spine

FOOT TECHNIQUES

Reflex ball on the sides of your foot
(p. 118)

Reflex ball on the ball of your foot, with your fingers wrapped around your heel
(p. 118)

Starting at the heel, thumb walk on the inside of the foot
(p. 150)

Continue to thumb walk on the inside of the foot, repositioning your hand if necessary
(p. 150)

HAND TECHNIQUES

Reflex ball on the side of
your thumb by the nail
(p. 117)

Reflex ball on the base
of your hand
(p. 117)

Thumb walk on the inside
edge of the hand
(p. 158)

CHRONIC FATIGUE SYNDROME

Chronic fatigue syndrome (CFS) is a debilitating medical condition with an unknown cause. Along with prolonged fatigue, sufferers often experience joint and muscle aches, sore throat, tender lymph nodes, and depression or other psychological problems. To help combat CFS, work the Pancreas, Adrenal gland, and Brain stem reflex areas.

Reflex areas: Brain stem, Pancreas, Adrenal glands

FOOT TECHNIQUES

Reflex ball on the edge of your foot along your big toe
(p. 118)

Foot roller on your inside arch
(p. 106)

Thumb walk on the inside arch of the foot
(p. 147)

HAND TECHNIQUES

Reflex ball on the heel
below your thumb
(p. 116)

Reflex ball on the edge of
your thumb by the nail
(p. 117)

Thumb walk on the heel
below the thumb
(p. 153)

COLD SORES OR CANKER SORES

Whether it's a cold sore (a blister caused by the herpes virus) or a canker sore (an ulceration of the mouth or lips), reflexology can help get rid of these nuisances more quickly. Feel carefully for the most sensitive area on the big toe or thumb.

Reflex area: Face

FOOT TECHNIQUES

Direct grip below the nail
of your big toe
(p. 123)

Thumb walk on the big toe
(p. 148)

HAND TECHNIQUES

Single-finger grip on your
thumb below the nail
(p. 121)

Thumb walk on the thumb
(p. 152)

CONSTIPATION

Constipation is a difficulty with bowel movements or unusually dry stool. It's most often caused by stress, not enough fiber or water intake, disruption of your regular diet, or pregnancy.

Reflex areas: Stomach, Colon, Small intestine, Pancreas, Gall bladder, Liver

FOOT TECHNIQUES

Foot roller from heel to mid-foot, while angling your foot to the inside, then center, then outside (p. 107)

Thumb walk on the lower arch and heel, from the inside to the outside (p. 146)

HAND TECHNIQUES

Reflex ball on the heel
of your hand
(p. 116)

Thumb walk on the palm
(p. 154)

Thumb walk on the
heel of the hand
(p. 155)

DEPRESSION

Depression is a feeling of sadness or hopelessness that lasts for an extended period of time. Use reflexology to help ease depression.

Reflex areas: Solar plexus/Diaphragm, Pancreas, Adrenal glands

FOOT TECHNIQUES

Foot roller on your arch
(p. 106)

Thumb walk between the
ball of the foot and the arch
(p. 144)

HAND TECHNIQUES

Pinch technique below
your thumb and each
of your fingers
(p. 122)

Reflex ball on the heel
below your thumb
(p. 116)

Single-finger grip on the
heel below the thumb
(p. 132)

DIABETES OR HYPOGLYCEMIA

Both diabetes and hypoglycemia relate to blood sugar levels. Diabetes occurs when your body has trouble burning up sugar because of an insufficient supply of insulin (a hormone produced by the pancreas), and hypoglycemia is a deficiency of sugar in the blood. You can use reflexology to help with circulatory problems and blood sugar stability by working the Pancreas reflex area.

Reflex area: Pancreas

FOOT TECHNIQUES

Foot roller on the upper arch with your foot angled toward the inside
(p. 107)

Thumb walk on the inner arch
(p. 147)

HAND TECHNIQUES

Reflex ball on the heel
below your thumb
(p. 116)

Thumb walk on the heel
below the thumb
(p. 153)

DIGESTIVE TROUBLE

Our digestive systems are a complex series of organs that are easily disrupted. You can use reflexology to make digestion easier.

Reflex areas: Stomach, Colon, Small intestine, Pancreas, Gallbladder, Liver

FOOT TECHNIQUES

Foot roller from your heel to the center of your foot, while angling your foot to the inside, then center, then outside
(p. 107)

Thumb walk from the heel to the center of the foot
(p. 147)

HAND TECHNIQUES

Reflex ball on your palm
(p. 116)

Thumb walk on the palm
(p. 154)

Thumb walk on the heel of
the hand
(p. 155)

DIZZINESS

Dizziness can result from any number of causes. Although it rarely signals a serious, life-threatening condition, dizziness can be disabling and incapacitating. Aging increases the risk of developing a condition that causes dizziness, one of the most common reasons older adults visit their doctors.

Reflex areas: Pituitary gland, Inner ear

FOOT TECHNIQUES

Single-finger grip on the center of your big toe (p. 121)

Pinch technique in the webbing between your toes (p. 122)

Thumb walk on the big toe (p. 148)

Single-finger grip in the webbing between the toes (p. 129)

HAND TECHNIQUES

Single-finger grip on the center of your thumb (p. 121)

Pinch technique in the webbing between your fingers (p. 122)

Single-finger grip on the center of the thumb (p. 132)

Single-finger grip in the webbing between the fingers (p. 131)

EARACHE

Most commonly found in children, pain in the ear is usually caused by infection and is most often a complication of an upper respiratory infection, such as a cold. Reflexology can help to lessen earache pain and make the infection go away sooner, and using these techniques regularly helps prevent chronic earaches in small children.

Reflex area: Ears

FOOT TECHNIQUES

Pinch technique in the webbing between your toes
(p. 122)

Single-finger grip in the
webbing between the toes
(p. 129)

HAND TECHNIQUES

Pinch technique in
the webbing between
your fingers
(p. 122)

Single-finger grip in the
webbing between the fingers
(p. 131)

EYE STRAIN/CATARACTS

Reflexology work can help to ease eye strain. In addition, it has been known to reduce the pain of cataracts.

Reflex area: Eyes

FOOT TECHNIQUES

Pinch technique in the
webbing between your toes
(p. 122)

Single-finger grip in the
webbing between the toes
(p. 129)

HAND TECHNIQUES

Pinch technique in
the webbing between
your fingers
(p. 122)

Single-finger grip in the
webbing between the fingers
(p. 131)

FEVER

Most frequently a symptom of infection, fevers can leave you laid up for days. You can use reflexology to reduce a fever.

Reflex area: Pituitary gland

FOOT TECHNIQUES

Single-finger grip on the center of your big toe
(p. 121)

Thumb walk on the big toe
(p. 148)

HAND TECHNIQUES

Single-finger grip on the
center of your thumb
(p. 121)

Single-finger grip on the
center of the thumb
(p. 132)

HANGOVER

The aftermath of drinking too much alcohol can result in headache, nausea, and other regrettable effects. To help ease this affliction, work various Head reflex areas by using the reflex ball on your fingertips and the foot roller and reflex ball on your toes; affect the Adrenal gland reflex area by rolling the ball on your lower palm.

Reflex areas: Head, Adrenal glands

FOOT TECHNIQUES

Foot roller on your toes
(p. 104)

Reflex ball on the first segment of your big toe
(p. 118)

Thumb walk on the toes
(p. 148)

HAND TECHNIQUES

Reflex ball on the first
segment of your thumb
(p. 113)

Reflex ball on the heel
below your thumb
(p. 116)

Thumb walk on the thumb
(p. 152)

Thumb walk on the fingers
(p. 152)

HEADACHE

Headaches have many different causes, and more than 40 million people in the United States experience chronic headaches. Whether you get headaches frequently or rarely, you can help decrease their severity by using reflexology.

Reflex areas: Head, Solar plexus

FOOT TECHNIQUES

Foot roller on your toes
(p. 104)

Reflex ball on the first
segment of your big toe
(p. 118)

Thumb walk on the toes
(p. 148)

HAND TECHNIQUES

Reflex ball on the first segment of your thumb (p. 113)

Reflex ball on the base of your thumb (try rocking the ball back and forth rather than rolling it in circles) (p. 115)

Thumb walk on the thumb (p. 152)

Thumb walk on the fingers (p. 152)

HEART PROBLEMS

The heart has a big job: keeping the blood circulating to carry nutrients, hormones, vitamins, antibodies, heat, and oxygen to our bodies' tissues as well as taking away waste materials. Focus your efforts on the Heart reflex area, but also apply pressure to the Solar plexus area, which will reduce stress and lower blood pressure, leading to a healthier heart.

Reflex areas: Heart, Solar plexus

FOOT TECHNIQUES

Foot roller on the ball of
your foot while angling
your foot to the inside
(p. 105)

Thumb walk on the ball
of the foot
(p. 144)

HAND TECHNIQUES

Reflex ball on the base
of your thumb
(p. 113)

Thumb walk at the
base of the thumb
(p. 153)

HEARTBURN

Heartburn, or acid reflux, happens when acid from your stomach trickles up into your esophagus due to a valve in your lower esophagus opening too frequently or not closing tightly enough. Sometimes caused by a hiatal hernia, frequent heartburn is called gastroesophageal reflex disease (GERD), and can cause a variety of symptoms such as difficulty swallowing and damage to your esophagus. Reflexology can help lessen the frequency of heartburn.

Reflex area: Solar plexus

FOOT TECHNIQUES

Foot roller on the ball of your foot, especially below the big toe and second toe (p. 105)

Thumb walk on the ball of the foot, especially below the big toe and second toe (p. 144)

HAND TECHNIQUES

Reflex ball on the base
of your thumb (rock the
ball back and forth
rather than roll it)
(p. 115)

Single-finger grip at the
base of the thumb
(p. 132)

HEPATITIS C

Hepatitis C is the inflammation of the liver caused by blood infected with the Hepatitis C virus. An estimated 3.9 million Americans have been infected with Hepatitis C, and most (but not all) go on to have chronic liver problems. You can use reflexology to help keep your liver healthy.

Reflex areas: Liver, Adrenal glands

FOOT TECHNIQUES

Foot roller on your arch
(p. 106)

Thumb walk on the arch
(p. 146)

HAND TECHNIQUES

Reflex ball on your
lower palm
(p. 116)

Single-finger grip on
the heel below the thumb
(p. 132)

Thumb walk on
the upper palm
(p. 153)

HIGH BLOOD PRESSURE

High blood pressure, or hypertension, is estimated by the American Heart Association to affect nearly one in three adults. High blood pressure increases the risk for kidney disease, heart disease, and stroke, some of the leading causes of death in the United States. To help lower your blood pressure, regularly use the reflex ball and the foot roller to work the Solar plexus and the Kidney reflex areas in the center of your feet and hands.

Reflex areas: Solar plexus, Kidneys

FOOT TECHNIQUES

Foot roller where the ball of your foot meets the arch (p. 105)

Foot roller on your arch (p. 106)

Thumb walk on the arch (p. 146)

Thumb walk from the ball of the foot to the upper arch (p. 144)

HAND TECHNIQUES

Reflex ball on the base
of your thumb (rock the
ball back and forth
rather than roll it)
(p. 115)

Reflex ball on your palm at
the base of the webbing
between your thumb and
index finger
(p. 116)

Thumb walk at the base of
the webbing between the
thumb and index finger
(p. 154)

INCONTINENCE

Although it's often not talked about, incontinence (loss of bladder control) affects 25 million adults in the United States, according to the National Association for Continence. Reflexology work on the Bladder as well as the Brain stem can help lessen an incontinence problem.

Reflex areas: Brain stem, Bladder

FOOT TECHNIQUES

Foot roller on your
lower arch
(p. 107)

Reflex ball on the edge
of your big toe
(p. 118)

Thumb walk on the inside
edge of the foot
(p. 150)

Thumb walk on the inside
edge of the big toe
(p. 150)

HAND TECHNIQUES

Reflex ball on the edge of
your thumb by the nail
(p. 117)

Reflex ball on the base
of your hand
(p. 117)

Thumb walk on the inside
edge of the thumb
(p. 158)

Thumb walk on the base
of the hand
(p. 158)

INFERTILITY

Reflexology is in standard use at some fertility clinics, as many women believe it has helped them conceive. Even if you're not trying to conceive, hormones produced by the reproductive glands impact virtually every part of the body.

Reflex areas: Ovaries/Testicles, Uterus/Prostate

FOOT TECHNIQUES

Rotate on a point on the inside of your ankle
(p. 125)

Rotate on a point on the outside of your ankle
(p. 125)

Rotate on a point on the ankle
(p. 138)

Thumb walk on the ankle
(p. 151)

HAND TECHNIQUES

Rotate on a point
on your wrist
(p. 125)

Rotate on a point
on the wrist
(p. 139)

INSOMNIA

Insomnia is the inability to fall asleep or stay asleep long enough to feel rested. Reflexology can help ease overall body stress, making it easier to sleep, and focusing specifically on the Solar plexus reflex area can help with insomnia.

Reflex area: Solar plexus

FOOT TECHNIQUES

Foot roller in between
the ball of your foot
and the arch
(p. 105)

Thumb walk on the ball
and upper arch of the foot
(p. 144)

HAND TECHNIQUES

Reflex ball at the base
of your thumb
(p. 115)

Single-finger grip in the
webbing between the thumb
and the index finger
(p. 131)

KIDNEY PROBLEMS

The chief filters of the urinary system, the kidneys help regulate fluid in the body. Reflexology has been shown to improve blood flow to the kidneys, helping guard against diabetes and other kidney problems.

Reflex area: Kidneys

FOOT TECHNIQUES

Foot roller on your arch
(p. 107)

Thumb walk on the lower arch
(p. 145)

HAND TECHNIQUES

Reflex ball on your
lower palm
(p. 116)

Direct-grip technique on
your lower palm
(p. 123)

Thumb walk on the
lower palm
(p. 154)

MEMORY LOSS

Loss of memory can affect anyone, but is most often associated with the aged. Use reflexology to help improve your memory.

Reflex area: Head/Brain

FOOT TECHNIQUES

Reflex ball on the first segment of your big toe (p. 118)

Foot roller on your toes (p. 104)

Thumb walk on the toes (p. 148)

HAND TECHNIQUES

Reflex ball on the first
segment of your thumb
(p. 113)

Thumb walk on the thumb
(p. 152)

Thumb walk on the fingers
(p. 152)

MENOPAUSE

This "life change" in women is usually accompanied by hot flashes, weight gain, feelings of weakness, and sometimes mental depression. Using reflexology can help ease these symptoms, especially hot flashes. Apply pressure to the heel's and palm's Uterus reflex area by using the reflex ball on your lower palm and the foot roller on your heel.

Reflex area: Uterus

FOOT TECHNIQUES

Foot roller on the center
of your heel
(p. 108)

Thumb walk on the heel
(p. 147)

HAND TECHNIQUES

Reflex ball on your
lower palm
(p. 116)

Thumb walk on the
lower palm
(p. 154)

MENSTRUATION

Painful periods not only reduce the quality of life for women, they sometimes make it impossible to go about daily life. Chronic cramping in the lower abdomen during periods even has a name—dysmenorrhea—and can worsen when you're under stress. With reflexology work, you can help ease the discomfort of periods.

Reflex areas: Uterus, Ovaries

FOOT TECHNIQUES

Rotate on a point on the inside of your ankle
(p. 125)

Rotate on a point on the outside of your ankle
(p. 125)

Rotate on a point on the ankle
(p. 138)

Thumb walk on the ankle
(p. 151)

HAND TECHNIQUES

Rotate on a point
on your wrist
(p. 125)

Rotate on a point
on the wrist
(p. 139)

MIGRAINE HEADACHE

Migraine headaches are chronic, intense headaches that can last up to 72 hours and are often accompanied by nausea or visual disturbances. These techniques can also help ease the pain associated with cluster headaches, trigeminal neuralgia, vascular disorders, and post-traumatic head pain.

Reflex area: Head

FOOT TECHNIQUES

Foot roller on your toes
(p. 104)

Reflex ball on the first segment of your big toe
(p. 118)

Thumb walk on the toes
(p. 148)

HAND TECHNIQUES

Reflex ball on the first segment of your thumb (p. 113)

Modify the direct-grip technique by sliding the flat of your thumb down your finger while stretching your finger to the side (p. 123)

Thumb walk on the thumb (p. 152)

Thumb walk on the fingers (p. 152)

PREMENSTRUAL SYNDROME

PMS is characterized by physical, psychological, and emotional disturbances brought on by changing hormonal levels after ovulation, normally ending with the onset of your period.

Reflex areas: Uterus, Ovaries

FOOT TECHNIQUES

Rotate on a point on the outside of your ankle
(p. 125)

Rotate on a point on the inside of your ankle
(p. 125)

Rotate on a point on the ankle
(p. 138)

Thumb walk on the ankle
(p. 151)

HAND TECHNIQUES

Rotate on a point
on your wrist
(p. 125)

Rotate on a point
on the wrist
(p. 139)

SCIATICA

"Sciatica" is the term for lower back pain (around the sciatic nerve) that travels through the buttock and down one leg. The pain usually goes past the knee and may go farther to the foot, sometimes causing weakness in the leg muscles. To work the Sciatic nerve reflex area, use the reflex ball on your lower palm and the foot roller on your heel.

Reflex area: Sciatic nerve

FOOT TECHNIQUES

Foot roller on the center
of your heel
(p. 108)

Thumb walk on the heel
(p. 147)

HAND TECHNIQUES

Reflex ball on your
lower palm
(p. 116)

Thumb walk on
the lower palm
(p. 154)

SHOULDER PAIN

Minor shoulder problems often occur from over-exercise or simply normal use. Reflexology is an easy way to help ease shoulder pain.

Reflex area: Shoulders

FOOT TECHNIQUES

Foot roller below your pinky toe while angling your foot to the outside (p. 105)

Thumb walk on the ball of the foot below the little toe (p. 149)

HAND TECHNIQUES

Reflex ball below
your little finger
(p. 115)

Thumb walk on the palm
below your little finger
(p. 155)

SINUSITIS

Sinusitis is the inflammation of the tissue lining of your nose and other sinus passages. Often caused by a cold or allergies that lead to an infection, sinusitis can result not just in a stuffy nose, but in headache; neck pain; earache; pain in the teeth, jaws, and cheeks; and eyelid swelling.

Reflex areas: Sinus passages, Adrenal glands

FOOT TECHNIQUES

Foot roller on your toes
(p. 104)

Foot roller on your arch
(p. 106)

Thumb walk on the toes
(p. 148)

Thumb walk on the arch
(p. 145)

HAND TECHNIQUES

Reflex ball on your fingers
(p. 114)

Single-finger grip on
your palm, feeling for the
most sensitive area
(p. 121)

Single-finger grip
on the palm
(p. 132)

Thumb walk on the fingers
(p. 152)

SORE THROAT

Most sore throats are caused by minor illness. Try using reflexology to ease this common occurrence.

Reflex area: Throat

FOOT TECHNIQUES

Foot roller on your toes
(p. 104)

Thumb walk on the big toe
(p. 148)

HAND TECHNIQUES

Reflex ball on the second
segment of your thumb
(p. 113)

Reflex ball on the heel of
your hand below the thumb
(p. 116)

Thumb walk on the thumb
(p. 152)

STOMACHACHE

Many things can lead to an upset stomach, from eating too quickly to stress. Stomachaches can be made worse by smoking, stress, excessive drinking of alcohol, and certain medications.

Reflex area: Stomach

FOOT TECHNIQUES

Foot roller on your upper arch while angling your foot to the center and then to the outside
(p. 106)

Thumb walk on the arch
(p. 145)

HAND TECHNIQUES

Reflex ball on the heel
of your hand below
your thumb
(p. 116)

Thumb walk on the heel of
the hand below the thumb
(p. 154)

STRESS

The American Psychological Association estimates that 75 to 90 percent of all visits to a doctor's office are due to a stress-related ailment. Sometimes we can't escape stress, but reflexology can help.

Reflex area: Solar plexus

FOOT TECHNIQUES

Foot roller in between
the ball of your foot
and the arch
(p. 105)

Thumb walk on the ball
and upper arch of the foot
(p. 144)

HAND TECHNIQUES

Pinch technique below
your thumb
(p. 122)

Reflex ball at the base
of your thumb
(p. 115)

Single-finger grip in
the webbing between the
thumb and index finger
(p. 131)

ULCER

Usually caused by an infection, an ulcer is a sore in the lining of your gastrointestinal tract, made worse by the acidic nature of the stomach and by stress. Symptoms of an ulcer can include nausea, vomiting, pain in the abdomen, and bloody stool.

Reflex area: Solar plexus

FOOT TECHNIQUES

Foot roller in between
the ball of your foot
and the arch
(p. 105)

Thumb walk on the ball
and upper arch of the foot
(p. 144)

HAND TECHNIQUES

Reflex ball on the base
of your thumb (rock back
and forth rather than roll)
(p. 115)

Single-finger grip in the
webbing between the
thumb and index finger
(p. 131)

Self Techniques

FINDING A REFLEXOLOGY TECHNIQUE THAT'S RIGHT FOR YOU is essential to making sure that you get the results you want and having the motivation to keep it up. Get comfortable and work through all of the reflex ball techniques, foot roller techniques, and manual techniques on the pages that follow to discover which ones work best for you. The hands are the most convenient site for reflexology work. They are easily accessible, which comes in handy when dealing with a chronic condition (such as hay fever) that needs a lot of continual work. The feet, however, offer a broader surface for pinpointing the appropriate reflex areas.

Initially, your foot or hand may feel stiff or tight. You may not feel that much is happening. Perhaps you'll enjoy the experience immediately or maybe take a while to develop a feel for it, as you may not be accustomed to spending so much time with your own hand or foot! To pique your interest, try this experiment. As you work, imagine yourself exploring a new sense, one seldom visited. Each and every pressure-sensing area of the hand or foot awakens a feeling of control over one's health. Not only will you relieve the tension of the day and begin to relax, but you will gain a foothold on becoming less stressed in the future.

Foot Roller

LET THE GOOD TIMES ROLL! Using a foot roller is a simple and easy way to get into reflexology. The foot roller is an invaluable tool for stimulating circulation throughout the feet, helping flush out excess fluids and toxins; but best of all, it makes your feet feel good!

Feet should feel good. Feet that feel bad are a product of overstress. Once you become familiar with using a foot roller, you'll be able to break up your individual patterns of stress, relaxing your feet so that they feel good all

What's Your Goal?

* If your goal is a general relaxation response for your body, use a gentle, slow, and easy rolling motion with light pressure. Use as frequently as desired and for as long as it's relaxing. Try it as a before-bed relaxant, an end-of-the-day wind-down, or to counter stress as it occurs (such as at work).

* If your goal is to rejuvenate your feet, target each foot's pattern of stress. Use the techniques discussed in this section to apply pressure generally (to counter an overall tired foot) or to a specific part of the foot that is stressed (such as an aching bunion). Use moderate pressure: enough to cause the foot to relax while still staying within your comfort zone. Use the foot roller frequently to break up the patterns of stress and keep them broken up.

* If your goal is to home in on a specific part of the body, focus on your technique application by doing it more frequently and for longer periods of time, carefully targeting your pressure for a maximum relaxation effect.

the time. Not only that, but relaxed feet help the whole body feel good. Practiced enough, foot-rolling will improve your overall health and reduce your potential for stress-related illnesses.

Time for your maiden voyage. Take a seat, slip on the reflexology socks, and get out the foot roller. Sit back, relax, and let the foot roller fly under the sole of your foot.

When you feel like taking a break, take your foot out for a test drive by standing up and taking a few steps. Notice how each foot feels and see if they match. Hopefully, your "rolled foot" will feel more relaxed. Now try rolling the other foot.

If you don't have your foot roller handy, you can also use a dowel rod, a couple of golf balls in a knotted sock, or other similar objects.

With a foot roller, you can relax your foot even with a small investment of time. As you use the roller, time yourself to see how long it takes to get that good feeling, and try to determine how long it lasts. Then come up with a strategy to continue that good feeling all day by setting a frequency for how often to use the roller to "take a load off."

If you would like to pursue more of a focused effort toward specific health goals (rather than general relaxation), take a look at the bottom of your reflexology sock–clad foot. The socks offer guides to stress patterns. A pattern of upper back and neck stress, for example, resides in the ball of your foot and your toes. Try rolling these areas of first one foot and then the other to gauge your upper back and neck stress. Notice the difference (if any) between the two. The foot that is more stressed may be the better foot for accessing your back and neck areas. Go on rolling that foot, seeing if you can make your upper back and neck feel more relaxed.

Be aware of how your foot feels as you roll over various areas. Consider how different areas feel—what feels good, and what doesn't? If an area feels good, work it more to relax your foot. If an area feels stressed, compare the location of the stressed part of your foot with the reflexology chart on the sock. Think about whether this matches your own health observations as well as observations by health care professionals.

Pick out some target areas according to what feels good or which health interests you'd like to pursue based on the reflex areas indicated on the reflexology chart. Use the techniques on the following pages that focus on these target areas. Once again, notice how long it takes to get that good feeling, and set a frequency (even if it's a general one) for rolling your feet throughout the day.

Always be aware of the potential for overwork, however, when using a hard object such as a foot roller. If, after reflexology work, the area feels sensitive in general or to the touch, it may be overworked. Let it rest for a few days. When you return to reflexology work, do so less frequently and for shorter periods of time. Wear a sock to reduce sensitivity. And make sure not to leave the roller where you or others may trip on it!

Check out the Introduction

for in-depth instructions on

how to find the techniques

that are right for you.

TOES

Place your foot on the foot roller and put the heel of your other foot on the top of your big toe. This will put more weight on the roller, giving you more control over it. You'll also be able to more accurately direct where pressure is applied. Roll slowly back and forth over the center of the big toe. Turn your heel slightly outward, allowing you to exert pressure on the outer edge of your big toe. Then turn your heel to the inside, exerting pressure on the inside of your big toe.

Move on, repositioning the heel of your foot over your middle toes, then your smaller toes. Roll each area for several minutes, turning your heel outward, then inward.

BALL OF THE FOOT

Start by simply rolling the foot roller back and forth over the surface of the ball of your foot while seated. ① Press down with your leg to exert more pressure. To cover the ball of the foot more fully, turn your foot to the inside, roll, and exert pressure. Then angle your foot to the outside and roll. ②

Now try working this part of the foot with a variation to get more pressure when rolling. Cross one leg over the other and then roll the foot roller back and forth over the surface of the ball of your foot, turning your foot first to the outside and then the inside.

UPPER ARCH

Place the foot roller under your arch. Roll from the edge of the ball to the center of the arch. **1** Press down with your leg to create more pressure. Turn your foot to the inside and roll, **2** then to the outside and roll. **3** Try crossing your legs to apply more pressure.

LOWER ARCH

Move the foot roller into the lower arch. Roll the center, ①
inside, ② and outside ③ ④ of the arch. Experiment with
exerting more pressure by rolling while pressing down with your
leg and then by crossing one leg over the other.

HEEL

Position the foot roller under your heel. **1** While rolling the foot roller, turn your foot first to the inside **2** and then to the outside. **3** If the roller tends to slip away, try crossing your legs, exerting more pressure and control over the roller.

Reflex Ball

DON'T LEAVE HOME WITHOUT IT—the reflex ball, that is. At least, that was the opinion of a certain five-year-old, who insisted on turning the car around to go home for "his" golf ball. As the story was told to us, it was the first his parents knew about the child's use of a reflex ball technique to ease his migraine headaches.

This speaks to the ease of using the reflex ball and its great advantage in addressing health concerns. It's small. It's portable. It's easy to use. And the

What's Your Goal?

* If your goal is a general relaxation response for your body, use a slow rolling motion with light pressure. Use as frequently as desired and for as long as it's relaxing. The reflex ball is easy to take with you, so it's perfect to use throughout the day to counter stress as it occurs.

* If your goal is to rejuvenate your hands, focus on the specific part of your hand that feels tired, and apply the reflex ball to counter overuse. Use moderate pressure: enough to cause your hand to relax while still staying within your comfort zone. Use frequently to break up the patterns of stress and keep them broken up.

* If your goal is to impact a specific part of your body and/or a specific health concern, the reflex ball is for you, thanks to its ability to target specific reflex areas coupled with the ease of frequent use. You'll want to use the reflex ball frequently enough to break up the pattern of stress. Give yourself time to learn the different reflex areas—some of which are pinpoint—and apply steady pressure.

hands are always accessible. Such a combination provides plenty of potential for success. Frequency counts in reflexology, and using the reflex ball means being able to easily work every part of the hand with the pressure needed for results.

Using a reflex ball provides many benefits: improved circulation, happy hands, and a way to tap into the body's natural resources for wellness. A reflex ball strategy allows you to interrupt patterns of stress and compensate for hardworking hands. Relaxed hands make the whole body feel good, and practiced enough, reflex ball techniques will result in improved health and a lessened potential for stress-related illnesses.

The reflex ball has a mind of its own! It even squirts out of our hands (sending our cats running for cover). The techniques in this chapter are designed for ball control.

In general, to use a reflex ball (which is simply a golf ball) cup it in your hand, press it against your other hand or a foot, and roll. Holding the ball in place is important both to keep it in control and effectively apply pressure, especially when targeting specific reflex areas. Be aware that it is easier to overwork an area with the reflex ball than with manual techniques. (Overwork has occurred when a touch to the area feels like a bruise.) Be conscious of your individual response to the pressure exerted by the ball, and choose a level of pressure according to your comfort level. If overwork does occur, let the area rest for a few days. When you begin again, use less pressure and/or work for less time to avoid future problems. While good for self-help, using the reflex ball to work on another person is not suggested. Problems can result from the combination of the ball's hard surface and too much pressure, and it's hard to gauge the results of the applied pressure on someone else.

Ready to roll? Get out the reflex ball, sit comfortably, and pull on the reflexology gloves. Rest one hand in your lap, palm up, with the other hand on top and the ball in between. Roll the reflex ball between your hands, covering both the fingers and palms.

Take a break and wiggle your fingers to test how each hand feels. (Since rolling the ball affects both hands, the difference between the two hands may not be as great as the difference you felt with the foot roller and your feet.) Go on rolling the ball between your hands, taking note of how long it takes to make your hands feel good and how long it lasts. Then establish a frequency for how often to use the reflex ball throughout the day.

Consider how different areas on your hand feel as you roll over them— what feels good, and what doesn't? If an area feels good, work it more to relax your hand. If an area feels stressed, the corresponding area of your body may need reflexology work. Compare the location of the stressed part of your hand with the reflexology chart on the glove. Think about whether this matches your own health observations as well as observations by healthcare professionals. A lower back or digestive stress pattern, for example, is pictured in the heels of the hands. To gauge your stress in this area, try rolling these parts of the hands, experimenting to see if you can make your lower back feel more relaxed. Try taking off the glove and rolling the ball on your bare hand to see if this works better for you.

Time yourself. Once again, notice how long it takes to make this area of your body feel better, and set a frequency (even if it's a general one) for using the reflex ball throughout the day. Develop a strategy for an all-day good feeling!

Since the flat surface of your hand is more readily accessible, you'll be able to target reflex areas on your hands more easily than you did on your feet. Pick out some target areas based on what feels good or on what health interests you'd like to pursue as indicated by the reflex areas on the chart. Use the instructions on the following pages to home in on these target areas. Once again, notice how long it takes to get that good feeling, and set a frequency (even if it's a general one) for rolling your hands throughout the day. Try keeping the reflex ball close at hand—on your desk, in the car, or by the TV; or take it with you in a purse or bag. And keep on rolling!

To better home in on your body's problem spots, try using the hands-on techniques in the next section.

REFLEX BALL TECHNIQUES

THUMB

To work the thumb, hold the ball with your index and middle fingers, positioning it as shown. ① Once in this position, pressing the ball with the thumb of your "working" hand controls the ball and creates pinpointed pressure. Now that you have a stable working surface, move your working hand to roll the ball across your thumb. Cover the length of the thumb with succeeding passes, repositioning your working hand as needed. ② Also try using the ball on the tip of your thumb. ③

FINGERS

Cup the reflex ball in your working hand, wrapping your four fingers around the finger to be worked. **1** The four fingers help to hold the ball in place and to create the desired amount of pressure. To generate more pressure, press with these fingers. To lessen pressure, loosen the grip of these fingers. Roll the ball over your index finger. Make succeeding passes until the length of the finger has been covered. Then continue with each remaining finger. **2**

UPPER PALM

To work your upper palm, begin by cupping the ball in your working hand. Place the ball at the base of your thumb and wrap your fingers around it. **1** Roll the ball back and forth, covering the joint and adjusting pressure by pressing with the fingers of your working hand. Reposition the ball below the index finger. **2** Roll the ball around the palm and into the trough between the knuckles and below your index and middle fingers. Again, lessen or increase pressure by adjusting the pressure of your working hand. Go on to work the knuckles below the middle, ring, and little fingers. **3**

LOWER AND CENTER PALM

The palms of both of your hands can be worked at the same time. Hold the reflex ball as shown, and roll it throughout the center of your palms, pressing with the fingers that are resting on the back of the hand to create more or less pressure. **1** Now try resting the ball in the heel of your hand below the thumb. Clasp your hands together, interlinking your fingers. **2** Roll the ball over this surface. Move on, positioning the ball lower on the heel of the hand and rolling here as well. **3**

OUTSIDE OF THE HAND

Cup the ball in the palm of your working hand, wrapping your fingers around your thumb (but this time without your thumbs touching). **1** Roll the ball, pressing with the fingers to create the desired pressure. Reposition your hand and the ball to further work the fleshy edge **2** and outside of the thumb. **3**

THE FOOT

The reflex ball is also an excellent tool for working certain areas of your foot. To work your toe, hold it in place with your hand. Then cup the ball in the palm of your other hand and roll it over the surface. **1** For the outside of the foot, steady the foot with your holding hand. Place the ball on the side of your foot and roll. **2** Make several passes. Reposition the ball as shown. **3** Wrap the fingers of your working hand around your foot to hold the ball in place and regulate pressure. Roll the ball, continuing to make several passes. Then reposition the ball and roll once again.

Hands-On Techniques

GET TO KNOW YOUR HANDS AND FEET with hands-on techniques. Learning manual techniques can take time, but there's nothing better for figuring out where your stressors are located. Tapping into the sensory-rich system of your hands and feet allows you to feed messages of relaxation into the stress mechanism and gather direct feedback about what parts of your hands or feet are stressed. Because you'll actually be able to feel the tension, manual techniques are an easy, straightforward way to reach reflex areas. So let's take a tour of hands-on techniques.

Slip on a glove and leave your other hand free to do the work. To apply a complete reflexology session to your hand, the goal is to make contact with

What's Your Goal?

* If your goal is to achieve an overall relaxation response, you'll want to apply techniques to your whole hand or foot.

* If your goal is to bring life back into your tired hands or feet, consider your level of tension. Flex your hand or rotate your foot, and decide what parts feel stressed, tight, or even painful. (In fact, your entire foot or hand may feel stressed.) Target the stressed areas with the techniques in this section.

* If your goal is to influence certain body parts and functions, these hands-on techniques allow you to target specific reflex areas. To create a reflex effect, give yourself time to learn the different reflex areas, some of which are pinpoint. Time your efforts and set a frequency to get results.

each area on the reflexology glove. Use the techniques on the following pages to make contact and exert pressure, going through all the reflex areas on one hand and then the other. As you go, consider what each area feel likes and compare the reflex areas on the first hand with their corresponding areas on the second hand. If an area on one hand is more sensitive than its counterpart, that side of your body may be under more stress than the other.

Next, slip on your reflexology sock and try working through all of the areas on your foot with the same techniques. Try to make contact with each area on the reflexology sock to give yourself a complete session. As you make contact and exert pressure, consider what the area feels like. Go on to the other foot, comparing the areas on this foot with the other.

Areas on the feet will be deeper than on the hands. Take care not to over-stress your working thumb or fingers!

Take care not to overwork your "working" hand by applying techniques longer than you're comfortably able. Switch to another technique if your hands feel strained. Also, some techniques may cause your fingernails to dig into the skin. Keep an eye out for fingernail marks on your hands and feet, and trim your nails or modify your grip as neccessary.

To apply these techniques to someone else's hands or feet, see Chapter 3: Techniques for Others

HANDS-ON TECHNIQUES

SINGLE-FINGER GRIP TECHNIQUE

Single-finger grip techniques are an easy way to work many parts of the hands and feet. Start by placing the tip of your index finger in the center of the thumb. **1** Apply pressure several times. Also try this technique in the heel of the hand below the thumb by curling your index finger into this fleshy part of the hand. **2** Your target is halfway along the long bone and slightly toward the webbing of the hand. Exerting pressure with the flat of the thumb works well in other parts of the hand, too. Give it a try by resting your thumb on top of the other thumb. **3** Press. Reposition your thumb; press again. Also try this on the palm of your hand.

1

2

3

HANDS-ON TECHNIQUES

PINCH TECHNIQUE

The webbing of the hands and feet provides a great opportunity to reach certain reflex areas that reflect body parts that are commonly stressed. Try this technique by placing the flats of your index finger and the thumb of your working hand in the webbing of your other hand. **1** Press several times. Reposition your hand by placing the flats of your finger and thumb in another portion of the webbing and press again. Go on to try this technique on the webbing between each of your other fingers **2** and the webbing between your toes. **3**

1

2

3

DIRECT-GRIP TECHNIQUE

Almost any part of your hand's palm or your foot's sole can be worked with the direct-grip technique. To try this technique, place the flat of your thumb on the sole of your foot and apply pressure. ① Try applying pressure to various areas on your foot, and then move on to your hand and try this technique there. Rest the flat of your thumb on the palm of your hand and press. ② Try moving your hand from side to side. (But be aware of the impact of your thumbnail on your palm.) Move on to other parts of your hand.

MULTIPLE-FINGER GRIP TECHNIQUE

For this technique, the tips of all four fingers are used to apply pressure across a wide area. First try this technique on the top of your foot. Rest your fingertips in the trough between the long bones. **1** Press several times. Go on to each trough. As you go, experiment with different angles and levels of pressure. Now try this technique on your hand by resting your fingertips in each trough and exerting pressure. **2** Try moving your hand from side to side and experimenting with other parts of your hand and foot.

ROTATING ON A POINT

To try rotating on a point, begin by resting your fingertip in the crease where your foot meets the ankle on the outside. **1** Exert pressure at your fingertip while turning your foot clockwise several times, drawing circles in the air with your big toe. Then turn your foot in a counter-clockwise direction several times. Reposition your fingertip as you try this technique at various spots around the ankle. Move your hand so that the flat of the thumb is approximately halfway between the ankle bone and the edge of the heel on the inside. **2** Press lightly with the thumb and turn the foot. To apply this technique to your hand, rest your finger-tip on your wrist. **3** Press gently with your working hand and move the other hand in a circle, first clockwise and then counter-clockwise.

1

2

3

3

Techniques for Others

THE FIRST RULE OF CREATING AN ENJOYABLE REFLEXOLOGY EXPERIENCE for someone else is to be in touch with the recipient's reaction to your work. What the recipient says and does are your cues to continue your work or find a better approach. As you work, ask "How does that feel?" If the answer is something like, "Good," or "It hurts a little, but feels good," then what you are doing is working—remember it for next time! If the response is "It hurts, and feels bad," use a lighter touch or a different technique. You should never be causing pain.

As you try the techniques and work the areas described in this chapter, you might notice that some people enjoy a particular technique no matter where it's applied, while others respond positively to certain techniques applied to particular reflex areas (use the socks or gloves to figure out if the individual's pattern of stress matches a reflex area). Remember, not only will you want to adjust your target areas and techniques, you will also want to adjust your pressure level, the length of time you apply the technique, and how frequently you apply it to find the mix that's right for your reflexology buddy. You should always be aware of how the recipient is responding to what you do, and be ready to make adjustments as your work progresses or as stress factors enter the individual's life.

Grip Techniques

GRIP TECHNIQUES ARE QUICK AND EASY ways to use reflexology to lower overall body stress, ease tired hands and feet, and target specific reflex areas. With grip techniques, you use your fingertip (or fingertips) to press a part of the foot or hand, then move to a new place and press again. When paired with the reflexology socks or gloves, they serve to create an uncomplicated and straightforward workout approach.

Because we all know how to grasp something, there is no new method to learn for the grip techniques. Focus instead on experimenting with exerting different levels of pressure with the tip of your finger or thumb as you explore the techniques. See what level of pressure applied repeatedly most relaxes your

What's Your Goal?

* If your goal for the individual is a general relaxation response for his or her whole body, use a very light touch as you apply these techniques.

* If your goal is to rejuvenate the individual's hands or feet, attempt to target the patterns of stress. Begin by using medium pressure, staying aware of his or her response. Try to find the proper amount of pressure to cause the hand or foot to relax.

* If your goal is to trigger a relaxation effect in a specific part of the body, you'll want to make a focused effort: spend more time doing it, do it more frequently, and consider the level of pressure that's most effective.

reflexology buddy. Remember, always begin reflexology work on another by pressing lightly. Don't press with your full strength!

As you go, take note of what parts of your reflexology buddy's hands or feet are stressed. If you're using the reflexology gloves or socks, note how these stressed areas relate to the reflex areas. Pick out some target areas based on which areas feel stressed or what health concerns your buddy would like to pursue. Use the techniques on the following pages to focus on these target areas, and maintain a steady pressure for a few seconds rather than pressing several times. Direct pressure such as this will create a painkilling effect in the corresponding part of the body.

Begin with the single-finger grip technique, in which your thumb will be working on the bottom of the foot or hand with your fingers resting on top. After you've tried the single-finger grip you'll be ready for the multiple-finger grip. Here you'll be using all of your fingertips at once to apply pressure across a broader area of the foot or hand. Finally, rotating on a point will show you how to pinpoint an area on your reflexology buddy's ankle or wrist.

Make sure your nails don't leave "chicken tracks" (our name for the impressions that nails leave on the feet or hands). Take care not to overly curl your fingers when applying the grip techniques, and keep your nails trimmed, so you don't leave a trail of nail prints as you work.

Once you've mastered the grip techniques, go on to the more advanced techniques of finger- and thumb-walking to give someone a full reflexology experience.

SINGLE-FINGER GRIP TECHNIQUES: FEET

BASE AND WEBBING OF THE TOES

Start by grasping the foot at the base of the toes. **1** Find the fleshy space between the toes and press lightly with your thumb and a fingertip. Press several times, increasing your pressure each time. Proceed to a new area (between two different toes) and repeat, **2** working your way across the foot. Get an idea of the individual's comfort level by asking him or her how it feels. If certain areas are sensitive or feel different, they may need more work.

BALL OF THE FOOT

Grasp the ball of the foot with your thumb on the sole and your fingers on top. **1** Find the spaces between the bones and press lightly, being careful not to dig your fingernail into the skin. Try this several times, gradually increasing pressure. Proceed to a new area and repeat, working your way slowly across the ball of the foot. **2** Again, ask about sensitivity.

Grasp the fleshy area to the outside of the foot by pressing your finger and thumb together. **3** Proceed up the foot and press. Ask about sensitivity.

SINGLE-FINGER GRIP TECHNIQUES: HANDS

WEBBING OF THE HAND

With your thumb on the top of the hand and your index finger on the palm, press your fingertips together through the webbing between the fingers several times. **1** Experiment by moving your fingers to another place in the webbing and pressing with your thumb. **2** Does the webbing under your fingertips feel different in different locations? If so, take note of which areas are more stressed and work them next time. Also try this technique on the fleshy outer edge of the hand.

THUMB AND PALM

Use your holding hand to hold back the individual's fingers. With your working hand, rest your index finger on the palm of the hand and your thumb on the top of the hand. **1** Gently press several times with the tip of your index finger. (Try to avoid digging your fingernail into the skin!) Move on, using this technique in the center of the thumb. **2** Try using different amounts of pressure in different places on the hand and see how it feels to your reflexology buddy.

MULTIPLE-FINGER GRIP TECHNIQUES: FEET

BASE OF THE TOES

Hold the foot steady with one hand as you rest your fingertips at the base of the toes. **1** Your fingers should be as close together as possible. Now press lightly several times, being careful not to dig your fingernails into the skin. Increase your pressure and ask your reflexology buddy how it feels. Reposition your fingertips and proceed to a new portion of the base of the toes. **2** Press repeatedly.

BALL AND UPPER ARCH

Wrap your hand around the foot as shown. **1** Reach around and rest the palm of your right hand on the top of the right foot with your fingers resting on the sole of the foot, and press gently with your fingertips. Then press a little harder as you ask your buddy how it feels. Try to get an idea of the person's comfort level. Proceed across the foot, lifting your arm up to allow yourself to apply more pressure as desired. **2**

TOP OF THE FOOT

Rest your fingertips lightly on the top of the foot with your thumb on the bottom. (Support the ankle with your other hand.) **1** Note that your fingertips fit conveniently between the long bones. Press several times, increasing your pressure as you go and asking your reflexology buddy how it feels. Try to avoid digging your fingernails into the skin. Work the area between each bone across the foot. **2**

MULTIPLE-FINGER GRIP TECHNIQUES: HANDS

PALM AND FINGERS

Hold back the fingers with your holding hand, and rest the finger-tips of your working hand on the palm. **1** Press with multiple fingertips gently. Experiment with differing levels of pressure while avoiding digging your fingernails into the skin. Increase your pressure and ask your reflexology buddy how it feels. Now move on to a different part of the palm and continue to press repeatedly.

You can also use the multiple-finger grip on each finger. **2** Press gently with your fingertips, then a little harder as you ask your buddy how it feels. Try to get an idea of the person's comfort level. Proceed to each finger, gauging your buddy's response as you go.

BACK OF THE HAND

The multiple-finger grip technique is especially good for the back of the hand. With your thumb on the palm of the hand and your fingers together on top, find the areas between the long bones in the hand. **1** Press gently several times as you move across the hand to each area. **2** When you get close to the thumb move your hand to the other side and grasp from the front. **3**

ROTATING ON A POINT TECHNIQUES

ANKLE

Cup the heel, wrapping your hand around the foot and resting your middle finger halfway between the ankle bone and the back of the heel. Wrap your other hand around the ball of the foot, and rotate the foot in a clockwise direction several times, drawing circles in the air. Then rotate the foot in a counter-clockwise direction several times.

WRIST

While holding the hand in place top side up, place the tip of your index finger on the top of the wrist with your thumb resting on the bottom. ① With your holding hand, grasp the upper hand and turn it in a clockwise direction, drawing circles in the air. Then turn it in a counter-clockwise direction. Pinpoint another area on the wrist and repeat. ②

1

2

Thumb- and Finger-Walking Techniques

"WALK" ALONG THE HANDS AND FEET with these techniques, which provide precise pressure by using the edge of the thumb or fingers as they "walk." Thumb- and finger-walking techniques are designed to maximize efficiency and effectiveness in applying pressure to the hands and feet. In reflexology, "efficiency" means covering a reflex area with the least amount of effort; "effectiveness" means hitting the points—being dead-on target in every reflex

What's Your Goal?

* If your goal is to achieve an overall relaxation response, apply these techniques to the entirety of both feet or hands using light pressure.

* If your goal is to bring life back into tired feet and hands, take note of the stressed parts as you go. Work through each foot and hand, focusing special attention on these parts.

* If your goal is to affect certain body parts or to address health concerns, thumb- and finger-walking techniques allow you to easily target specific reflex areas. Use the reflexology socks and gloves, and give yourself time to learn how to effectively apply pressure to individual reflex areas, some of which are quite small and can be difficult to pinpoint.

area. With a little practice, thumb and finger walking will be among your most useful tools in reaching these goals, because the interplay between the holding fingers and thumb will give you the ability to exert pressure on all of the varied surfaces of the hands and feet.

Thumb walking is achieved by bending your thumb at the first joint (the one closest to the tip of your thumb), and then taking small "steps" with it across the hand or foot. Pressure is increased or decreased by lifting or dropping your wrist, as this uses leverage to create pressure at the thumb's tip. Finger walking is most frequently used on the bony tops and sides of the feet. Either one finger or all fingers work the surface. Like thumb walking, the basis of the finger-walking technique is the bending of the working fingers at their first joints.

Before you begin thumb and finger walking on your reflexology buddy's feet and hands, give it a try on your own arm so you can get a feel for it first. Use the instructions that follow to practice thumb and finger walking.

Practice thumb and finger walking using the instructions that begin on the next page before you go on to the walking techniques that follow. }

Bend and unbend your thumb at the first joint while grasping it at the second joint to keep it steady. This movement is the basis of thumb or finger walking. **1**

Rest your hand on your leg and try this same move. Your thumb should "walk" forward. Continue to bend and unbend your thumb, taking small steps forward with each unbending motion. **2**

Now try practicing this technique on your arm. Rest your fingertips on the top of your arm with your thumb on your arm's underside. While keeping your fingers in place, bend and unbend your thumb against the under-side of your arm. As you unbend your thumb, take a small step forward. Practice walking your thumb in a forward direction. Keep your other fingers in place until your hand is stretched uncomfortably, then reposition them, continuing to keep them in place as your thumb walks. **3**

As you practice thumb walking, make sure you're only bending your thumb at the first joint! If you find that your thumb tires easily, you may be pressing with it instead of "walking" with it. Focus on creating leverage by dropping your wrist rather than pressing with your thumb. The same apples to finger walking.

Maintaining the position of your fingers, lower your wrist slightly. Do you notice that the tip of your thumb is now exerting more pressure? Now drop your wrist lower. Your thumb should be exerting even more pressure. As you can feel, leverage is created by an interplay of the fingertips, wrist, and thumb tip. **4**

Practice the thumb-walking technique by walking along your arm. As you go, try to exert constant, steady pressure. This is most easily achieved by effective use of leverage as described in step 4. **5**

To finger walk, rest your index finger on the top of your hand, and work up the hand in between the bones, taking small "steps" while maintaining constant, steady pressure. **6**

Take care not to overwork your hands by applying techniques longer than you're comfortably able. If your hands become tired, switch to another technique. Make sure to give yourself time to learn the techniques and how best to make the most of the physical effort expended. Though they may take a little while to learn, these walking techniques will become one of the most valuable tools in your reflexology arsenal.

4 **5** **6**

THUMB-WALKING TECHNIQUES: FEET

BALL

For this technique, your right hand will be your "working" hand while your left hand serves as the "holding" hand. With your left hand, pull the toes back slightly. This will steady the foot and position it to make a smoother surface for easier thumb walking. Note the troughs between the bones in the ball of the foot. Rest the thumb of your right hand at the base of a trough. **1** Dropping your wrist to create leverage, bend and unbend your thumb at the first joint to move it forward. Take small steps forward and exert constant, steady pressure. Move on to each trough and repeat. **2**

ARCH

Hold back the toes with your left hand. Following a straight path as shown by the arrows, move your right thumb forward, by bending and unbending at the first joint. **1** As you finish one path, reposition your thumb, drop your wrist to create pressure, and then move the thumb forward, tilting the foot if necessary. **2** By following the arrows, a systematic pattern of thumb walking is applied to the feet.

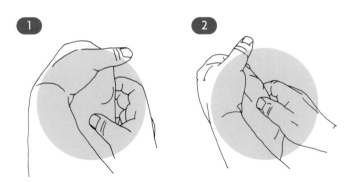

LOWER ARCH AND HEEL (INSIDE TO OUTSIDE)

Move your right hand to the bottom half of the foot while still using your left hand to hold back the toes. ❶ As your right thumb moves up the foot, note the tendon that runs up the ball of the foot on the inside of he arch (the big-toe side). Don't apply full pressure while moving over the tendon. Let up slightly with the left hand, so that the foot is not so tightly stretched. Create an appropriate amount of pressure at the tip of your thumb by raising and lowering the wrist of your right hand.

LOWER ARCH AND HEEL (OUTSIDE TO INSIDE)

Up until now, you've been using your left hand as your "holding" hand and your right hand as your "working" hand. Now we're going to switch it up! Using your right hand as holding hand, position the thumb of your left hand on the foot. Now move your thumb up the foot **1** and then toward the inside of the foot rather than the outside. **2** For the lower parts of the foot, try holding it at the heel rather than at the toes. **3** Even if you're not left-handed, the ability to use either hand as your working hand is worth developing because it will allow you to work all parts of the foot. It's also useful for giving your right thumb a rest!

THUMB-WALKING TECHNIQUES: FEET

TOES

Work the toes by wrapping your right hand (the holding hand) behind the toes. Rest the fingers of your left hand on top of those of your right hand. ❶ As the thumb of your left hand applies the thumb-walking technique, working in downward direction, your right hand serves as a backstop. Each toe is held in place by being pressed against your right hand. Keep this backstop in place as you apply the technique to each toe. ❷

BASE OF THE TOES

To work the base of the toes, pull down on the foot with your left (holding) thumb to smooth the fleshy base of the toes, while your left-hand fingers serve as a backstop for the toes. Rest the fingers of your right hand on top of those of your left hand. ❶ Rest your right-hand thumb at base of the toes, then walk it from the big toe to the little toe. ❷ You can also try changing hands so your left hand is the working hand and your right is the holding hand, working your way back up the base of the foot from little toe to big toe.

❶   ❷

INSIDE OF THE FOOT

Begin by holding the foot steady with your holding hand so that the foot's inside edge is accessible to your working thumb. **1** While cupping the heel with your working hand, begin thumb walking toward the big toe, moving the thumb in a forward direction. As you work, continuously reposition your working hand so that your thumb is not overstretched. **2** Continue up the side of the big toe. **3**

1

2

3

OUTSIDE OF THE FOOT

Cup the heel with your (right) holding hand. With your (left) working hand, rest your index finger under the ankle bone. **1** Now walk forward with your finger, tracing around the ankle bone. Next, hold the top of the foot with your right hand. Use the thumb of your left hand to thumb walk on the outside of the foot, repositioning your working hand as necessary. **2**

1

2

THUMB-WALKING TECHNIQUES: HANDS

FINGERS

With your holding hand, stretch the fingers back, beginning with the thumb, so that the hand is open. With your working hand, rest your fingers underneath the hand and place your thumb at the base of your buddy's thumb. **1** Raising your wrist to create leverage as necessary, bend and unbend your thumb at the first joint to move it around the thumb. **2** Take small steps and exert constant, steady pressure. Proceed in the same manner with each digit. **3**

UPPER PALM

While holding the fingers back with your holding hand, position the thumb of your working hand so that it rests on the bony joint below your buddy's thumb. **1** Now walk your thumb forward (away from the individual's thumb), making several passes. Move on to the bony joint below the index finger. **2** Work your way across the hand, working each joint as well as the trough between each finger. **3**

1

2

3

THUMB-WALKING TECHNIQUES: HANDS

LOWER PALM

To use the thumb-walking technique on the lower palm, begin in the fleshy part of the hand below the thumb. **1** With the fingers of your working hand resting on the back of the hand for leverage, walk your thumb down to the wrist. Reposition your thumb and make several passes, each time beginning at the padded part of the palm. **2** **3**

1

2

3

HEEL OF THE HAND

Hold back the fingers with your holding hand, and position your working thumb near the wrist. **1** Thumb walk down the wrist, making a series of passes to cover the area. To work just above the heel, position your working thumb above the heel of the hand below the index finger. **2** Holding the fingers back, thumb walk down the palm. Reposition your thumb and make several passes.

THUMB-WALKING TECHNIQUES: HANDS

TOP OF THE HAND

The top of the hand is a bony surface with troughs that form convenient working paths for your thumb-walking technique. Rest your working thumb at the base of the fingers, **1** and thumb walk along each bony trough. **2**

1   **2**

FINGERS

Rest your buddy's fingers on the fingers of your holding hand, and use the thumb of your holding hand to hold those fingers steady. With your working hand, begin at the base of the nail ① and work your way across the first finger, ② bending your thumb at the first joint and taking small steps. Move your holding thumb as necessary, and continue on to each finger.

① ②

THUMB-WALKING TECHNIQUES: HANDS

INSIDE OF THE HAND

To work the inside edge of the hand, first hold the thumb in a stationary position. With your working hand, use the thumb-walking technique to walk up the inside edge. **1** Reposition your hand as your thumb becomes stretched. Now go on to the inside edge of the thumb. **2**

FINGER-WALKING TECHNIQUES: FEET

DOWN THE TOP OF THE FOOT

Sit facing the soles of the feet of your reflexology buddy. With your left (holding) hand, hold the big toe in place and spread it and the next toe apart to more easily access the trough between the long bones. Place the thumb of your right hand on the ball of the foot and your index finger at the base of the toe on the top of the foot. **1** Using the finger-walking technique, move your index finger down the troughs of the foot, in between the bones. You can also try working the toes themselves. **2**

ACROSS THE TOP OF THE FOOT

Position your left hand so that you're holding the foot by the ankle. Rest the thumb of your right hand on the sole of the foot. Using all of the fingers of your right hand, work your way across the top of the foot. **1** Make sure you're bending the fingers only after the first joint! To work across the toes, use only two fingers, or as many as will fit. **2**

Desserts

JUST AS DESSERTS ARE A FAVORITE PART OF ANY DINNER, these "dessert" techniques may become the favorite part of a reflexology workout. These relaxation techniques are perfect for interspersing throughout a routine to ease sensitivity, warming up the hand or foot for hands-on techniques, or creating an overall feeling of comfort.

In general, the joints and other areas of the hand or foot are moved in one way and then another as your working hands quickly, rhythmically, and systematically create movement. Desserts can play an important role in mitigating tension caused by the day-to-day activities of the hands and feet. By relaxing the hands or feet and moving them in new directions, the desserts are

What's Your Goal?

* Desserts are created specifically to relax the hands and feet. Try using them before you start a routine to get the hand or foot warmed up and ready to be worked on.

* If your goal is to rejuvenate the hands or feet, try using the desserts throughout a reflexology session to break up stress patterns and make the hands and feet more comfortable. An all-dessert session will help breathe life back into those tired feet and hands.

* Using desserts can help achieve your reflex-effect goals by providing an overall sense of relaxation. In addition, specific reflex areas can be affected when the dessert is applied in a particular region, such as in the Lung press dessert.

perfect to use at the beginning of a reflexology workout to get your buddy ready for the rest of the techniques. Desserts are also a great way to give your own hands a break from the more rigorous techniques if you feel them getting tired while giving someone a reflexology session!

When practicing dessert techniques, take care not to overwork your hands or arms by applying them for longer than you're comforably able. Sometimes, a particular technique might not feel good to your reflexology buddy. If that's the case, stop doing it and move on to the next technique.

Desserts are perfect for introducing your children to reflexology. (Not surprisingly, children love these desserts too!) With many of the techniques, the foot or hand moves so quickly that it becomes blur. Kids often find it very entertaining to see their hand or foot "disappear" in such a manner.

To learn how to use the desserts in conjunction with the rest of the techniques for others, see Chapter 4: Reflexology Sessions.

FOOT DESSERTS

SIDE-TO-SIDE

The side-to-side technique is a universal favorite. Rest your hands on the sides of the foot. **1** While pressing lightly, rapidly move your hands back and forth with a pistonlike action, bringing the inside and then the outside of the foot toward you. Thus the foot is moved in a side-to-side motion. For a variation (called the hook-in-the-ankles technique), rest the heels of your hands where the foot meets the ankle on either side and move rapidly. **2**

FOOT-FLICKING

For the foot-flicking technique, the foot is moved rapidly up and down. Grasp the foot with your left (holding) hand around the ankle. **3** With your right hand, grasp the big toe at its base. Now quickly move the foot up and down.

FOOT DESSERTS

FOOT CIRCLES

Turning the foot in a circle is a simple, yet effective, technique. Hold the foot at the ankle with your left hand. With your right hand, grasp the ball of the foot with your thumb on the bottom and your fingers on the top. **1** Now turn the foot as if you were drawing a circle in the air with the big toe. Do this several times in both a clockwise and a counterclockwise direction.

LUNG PRESS

To do the Lung press dessert, grasp the ball of the foot with your right hand with the thumb on the underside of the toes and your fingers on the top of the foot. Then rest the flats of the fingers of your left hand on the ball of the foot. **2** Press forward with your left hand, then press gently back with your right hand. The effect is one of a soft push and squeeze on the Lung reflex area.

HAND DESSERTS

PULL TECHNIQUE

The pull technique provides a gentle traction to each finger and segment of the hand. While holding the hand at the wrist, grasp the full length of the finger with your working hand and pull gently. **1** At the same time, counter this movement by pulling in the opposite direction at the wrist. Hold for several seconds, and then go on to each finger and the thumb. For another easy hand dessert, simply bend and unbend each finger gently.

SIDE-TO-SIDE

This technique moves the joints of the digits in seldom experienced directions. Position the flats of both of your thumbs and index fingers on either side of your buddy's index finger at the joints. **2** While pushing with the thumb of your right hand, also push with the index finger of your left hand. Do this several times, creating a side-to-side movement of the finger. Move on to each finger and the thumb.

1

2

HAND DESSERTS

THE WALK-DOWN

The walk-down technique uses thumb walking to stretch the fingers. Hold the hand at the wrist to steady it. With your working hand, place your fingertips on the side of the finger and the flat of your thumb on the other side at the first joint. Now drop your wrist to place the finger in a stretched position. **1** Without moving your fingers, walk down the finger with your thumb by using the thumb-walking technique. Make several passes, then try on each finger.

THE PALM-ROCKER

To relax the whole hand, use the palm-rocker technique. Grasp the person's hand at the knuckles with both of your hands, with the flats of your index and middle fingers on the top and your thumbs on the palm. **2** Simultaneously push with your right thumb and your left fingers, then counter the movement by pushing with your left thumb and right fingers. Do this several times at each of the joints.

THE PALM-LEVER

Further relax your buddy's hand by using the palm-lever technique. With your right hand, grasp the top of the long bone beneath the index finger. With your left hand, grasp the base of this bone. The flats of your thumbs should be resting on the palm. Now push with the fingers of your right hand as you push with the flat of your left thumb. Now switch, pushing with the fingers of your left hand while pushing with the flat of your right thumb. Practice this several times on each of the long bones of the hand.

Reflexology Sessions

NOW THAT YOU'VE BECOME ACQUAINTED WITH SOME BASIC SKILLS, it's time to put them together into entire reflexology routines that work each part of the feet and hands. Not only will they rejuvenate the hands and feet, these routines will work each individual reflex area and produce overall relaxation for the entire body.

These sessions begin with desserts to relax the foot or hand, progress through the grip techniques, and then go on to the more advanced walking techniques. If you're focused on affecting reflex areas, note the reflex area being worked. If a part of the foot or hand is particularly sensitive, it might indicate that work in that reflex area is needed. Use the reflexology socks or gloves to better pinpoint these areas. The more often you repeat these workouts, the better your ability will be to notice new areas of the hands and feet that are stressed. If any technique or part of the foot or hand feels particularly good or stressed, remember it for next time—or apply some more work now!

Whole Foot Workout

THE FEET ARE A GREAT PLACE TO START your reflexology work on someone else. Though you may not be as familiar with the surface of the foot as you are with the hand, the foot offers you a wide surface to target specific reflex areas and practice your reflexology techniques. A reflexology session on the feet can also help relax the entire body of your subject, as these techniques will help improve circulation and counter overstress in this often-used part of the body.

Start by seating your buddy and yourself comfortably, positioned so that you are facing the soles of his or her feet. Check to see if there are any areas to be aware of, such as cuts or bruises. Cover these areas with a bandage and avoid touching them as you go. Now it's time for a workout!

For a reflexology session focused
more on a particular health
concern, see the Reflex Areas chapter
at the beginning of the book.

WHOLE FOOT WORKOUT

DESERTS

Side-to-side (p. 163)

2

Foot-flicking (p. 163)

3

Foot-circling (p. 164)

4

5

6

Lung press (p. 164)

Single-finger grip on the webbing
of the toes (p. 129)

Single-finger grip in the spaces
between the bones on the
ball of the foot (p. 130)

Reflex areas: Eye, Inner ear, Ear

Reflex areas: Chest/Lung, Solar
plexus/Diaphragm

GRIP TECHNIQUES *(continued)*

Single-finger grip on the fleshy outer edge of the foot (p. 130)

Reflex areas: Arm, Elbow

Multiple-finger grip on the base of the toes (p. 133)

Reflex areas: Eye, Inner ear, Ear

Multiple-finger grip on the ball and arch of the foot (p. 134)

Reflex areas: Chest/Lung, Liver/ Gallbladder (right foot), Stomach (left foot)

10

Multiple-finger grip on
the top of the foot, in the troughs
between the long bones (p. 135)

Reflex areas: Upper back, Shoulder

11

Thumb walk down the center and
side of each toe (p. 148)

Reflex areas: Head/Brain, Sinus, Neck

12

Thumb walk across the base of the
toes from one direction and
then the other (p. 149)

Reflex areas: Eye, Inner ear, Ear

WALKING TECHNIQUES *(continued)*

Thumb walk up the ball of
the foot (p. 144)

Reflex areas: Chest/Lung, Solar plexus,
Shoulder

Thumb walk from the mid-arch
to the ball of the foot (p. 145)

Reflex areas: Pancreas/Adrenal gland,
Kidney/Liver/Gallbladder (right foot),
Kidney/Stomach (left foot)

Thumb walk up the foot from
the bottom, and then diagonally
across (p. 146)

Reflex areas: Colon, Small intestine

GRIP TECHNIQUES

Rotate on a point on the inside
of the foot (p. 138)

Reflex area: Uterus/Prostate

WALKING TECHNIQUES

Thumb walk up the inside edge
of the foot (p. 150)

Reflex areas: Tailbone/Bladder/
Lower back, Spine

Finger walk around the outside
ankle bone (p. 151)

Reflex area: Sciatic nerve

WALKING TECHNIQUES *(continued)*

Thumb walk up the outside edge
of the foot (p. 151)

Reflex areas: Ovary/Testicle,
Knee/Leg, Elbow/Arm

Finger walk across the top of each toe
(p. 160)

Reflex areas: Face/Teeth/Jaw

Finger walk across the top
of the foot (p. 160)

Reflex areas: Chest/Lung, Upper back/
Shoulder

22

Finger walk down each trough (p. 159)

23

Lung press (p. 164)

24

Foot-circling (p. 164)

Reflex areas: Shoulder, Chest/Lung, Upper back

DESSERTS *(continued)*

 25

 26

Foot-flicking (p. 163)

Side-to-side (p. 163)

Whole Hand Workout

TIME TO EASE THOSE TIRED HANDS with the whole hand workout. Not only will this routine rejuvenate your reflexology buddy's hands, it will allow you to work each individual reflex area, relaxing the whole body.

The workout begins with desserts to relax the hand, and works through the grip techniques, focusing primarily on thumb walking to get the most out of your reflexology session. Start by seating your buddy and yourself comfortably, positioned so that you are side by side. Rest the hand on a pillow or folded towel. Make sure to check if there are any areas to be aware of, such as cuts or bruises. Avoid working these areas, and cover cuts with a bandage to avoid touching them. Ready? Let's go!

For a **reflexology session** focused more on a particular health concern, see the **Reflex Areas chapter** at the beginning of the book.

DESSERTS

Pull technique (p. 165)

Side-to-side (p. 165)

Walk-down (p. 166)

4

5

6

Palm-rocker (p. 166)

Palm-lever (p. 167)

Single-finger grip on the thumb (p. 132)

Reflex areas: Pituitary gland, Adrenal gland

GRIP TECHNIQUES (continued)

Single-finger grip on the webbing between the fingers (p. 131)

Reflex areas: Eye/Ear, Kidney, Arm, Elbow

Multiple-finger grip on the back of the hand (p. 137)

Reflex area: Upper back

WALKING TECHNIQUES

Thumb walk on the fingers (p. 152)

Reflex areas: Head/Brain/Sinus, Neck

10

Thumb walk on the base
of the fingers (p. 153)

Reflex areas: Lung, Heart

11

Thumb walk on the base
of the thumb (p. 154)

Reflex areas: Adrenal gland, Pancreas,
Kidney

12

Thumb walk on the heel
of the hand (p. 155)

Reflex areas: Liver, Gallbladder (right
hand), Stomach, Spleen (left hand)

WALKING TECHNIQUES *(continued)*

13

Thumb walk on the edge
of the thumb (p. 158)

Reflex area: Spine

GRIP TECHNIQUES

14

Rotate on a point on the wrist (p. 139)

Reflex areas: Ovary/Testicle,
Uterus/Prostate

WALKING TECHNIQUES

15

Thumb walk down the backs
of the fingers (p. 157)

Reflex areas: Head, Neck

Thumb walk on the top
of the hand (p. 156)

Palm-lever (p. 167)

Palm-rocker (p. 166)

Reflex areas: Upper back, Lympathic
system

DESSERTS *(continued)*

Walk-down (p. 166)

Side-to-side (p. 165)

Pull technique (p. 165)

Index

Index

Index

Notes

Notes